The Dash Diet: Lose Weight Quickly and Safely for Life

BENJAMIN TIDEAS

CONTENTS

PRAISE FOR THE DASH DIET

When I originally heard about The Dash Diet, it helped motivate me to keep going and lose the last of my pregnancy weight as my son got his driver's license. It has been a very long road. As for the motivation piece – yes it's easy to fall off the wagon – however, if you take it step by step, and get back to your eating plan, it will work. The Dash Diet isn't one of those crazy diets where your family has to hide the chocolate cake or lock up the refrigerator. It was just a nice, gentle way to get back to a weight I felt comfortable about. – Tammy, 55, Wichita, KS.

By eating the Dash Diet on a consistent basis and being more consistent with my exercising, I gradually lost 30 pounds over the first six months that I tried it. and am now continuing to stay fit. My cholesterol came down from 195 in 2002 to 135 today – something my doctor and I were very pleasantly surprised about. I'm not sure where I would be today without The Dash Diet, but I don't think I would be nearly as active as I am. – Will, 72, Clovis, CA.

I've really participating in the Dash program for the first time in my life. I never realized how strong the correlation between eating healthy and feeling healthy really is – I didn't think it would be so easy!!! I feel great and I think eating more balanced meals has helped to curb my sweet tooth. This is definitely something I should have started years ago. – Noah, 43, Boston, MA.

I suffered a heart attack before the age of 40, so for me, changing my lifestyle was an absolute must. I didn't want to become a burden to my family. As part of my cardiac rehab program, I went to a dietitian who prescribed The Dash Diet to me. In the first 5 months, I lost 40 pounds on The Dash Diet. I found the diet very easy to understand

and simple to follow without taking out the things I really loved– a big part of the reason I was so successful. There was even an online program offered at my place of employment. I began to track my results on the website and keep my progress recorded in one location. I have lost a total of 60 pounds and lowered my cholesterol in the process (from a total cholesterol of 267 to 137). Dash really is a piece of cake – you've got nothing to lose in giving it a try. – Rachael 37, Philadelphia, PA.

I think The Dash Diet is a fantastic program! During the course of the program I went from a size 14 to a size 8-10. I had put on some weight thanks to college eating plans and I never really worked to take it off – Dash changed that. When I talk to people I hear all the time "What type of diet are you on?" What I say to them is that I'm not on a diet –Dash has given me a whole new way of looking at food and learning what to eat. DASH leaves the choices up to me. Also, learning about portion sizes and healthy food options was a huge part of my success. Thanks Dash! Brittany, 28, Columbia, OH.

When I started this program I was 185 lbs. My blood pressure was 140/90 (pre-hypertensive). I began this program not knowing what results I would get, but I was committed to change my eating habits to improve my health. My father had a heart attack when I was in high school, so I knew I was susceptible to problems. About a month into the program I had lost about 10lbs. and my blood pressure had dropped on both sides almost 10 points. I have been able to maintain this with little effort. I think the most important thing is that this program is something I can live with and have passed on to my children and family. I have developed and adopted a new happy and healthier life. –Kurt, 34, New York, NY.

The first thing I did when I started The Dash Diet was focus on eating smaller portion sizes and more vegetables. It was a nice, slow way to start, but still I saw results pretty quickly. The weight felt like it came off really quickly and easily, with some pretty simple changes. – Blaine, 33, New York, NY.

INTRODUCTION

I'd like to personally thank you for reading this book, "The DASH Diet: Lose Weight Safely and Effectively for Life."

Losing weight has been a popular subject for years now, with society's continued desire for smaller waistlines and pants sizes. There's no doubt that there have been thousands of methods, hundreds of thousands of books written, and a million more articles on the internet. So how did you end up with another book on this subject? Perhaps you did some research and discovered The Dash Diet. Maybe you saw it on "Dr. Oz". Perhaps you were browsing the internet for a way to lower your blood pressure. You could have gotten a pamphlet from your doctor at your last checkup. Maybe your friends have tried it.

Whatever the reason, you're about to learn a simple, easy, and solid method of losing weight without giving up too much of your lifestyle. And that's what is important, right? Inside you'll find exactly what you've been looking for.

Also, don't forget to grab your FREE Bonus book via the link at the end!

So let's begin this journey!

WHAT IS THE DASH DIET?

The Dash Diet, short for Dietary Approaches to Stop Hypertension, is, in its simplest form, a meal plan. Originally designed as a technique for lowering blood pressure (hypertension), it has spiraled into a diet that has spawned popularity from the National Institute of Health, the USDA, private practices, and countless online news websites. It's remained the #1 Most Recommended Diet for four years in a row, according to the US News & World Report! The Dash Diet focuses on the kind of foods you eat, how much you eat, and how to balance your meal plan with the things you enjoy and the things you should put into your body. Unlike a lot of diets, The Dash Diet paces you, so you're not thrown into an unfamiliar world of cravings for those midnight double cheeseburgers. Not only is this dietary plan designed to help lower your blood pressure, and lose weight, but it also promotes a healthier lifestyle, keeping you on this beautiful planet that much longer. Focusing on proper fruits, veggies, nuts and greenery, you'll be left satisfied, thinner, and all around feeling like an Olympic champion!

It is also significant to note, that this isn't a diet where you will have to run all over the countryside to find one obscure health food market to purchase your new edibles. These ingredients that you will be consuming can be found in almost any grocery store or farmer's market! Balance is important in any aspect of your life, especially eating and cooking. That's why The Dash Diet was designed to include different food groups and diverse meals so that you're not chomping on the same head of lettuce you started on two weeks ago. Luckily, you won't be feeling like you've stepped up to a challenge only fit for those health nuts that lift weights fourteen times a day and run 730 miles a week. The Dash Diet allows you to start reaping the benefits of the diet immediately and work yourself up to those stricter tactics.

You don't have to jump into the water head first, you can put your feet in and try it out for a while before slipping a little further into the methods. Incorporate The Dash Diet into your snacks at first, instead of your breakfast, lunch, and dinner schedule. Start using it for breakfast, and keep your lunches and dinners the same until you're ready to transition to your breakfasts and lunches. Eventually, you can move to having all of your meals follow the diet plan. There's no limit to the way you can utilize the advantages of this healthy eating alternative, and that's part of the fun – you're allowed to be creative with it.

One of the biggest problems in dieting is satisfying your metabolism. Think about all the times you've tried those different meal plans, and they leave you feeling like you could go for a burrito. I don't know about you, but my goal when I sit down looking at a plate with something I'm about to digest, I expect it to be tasty, fulfilling, and leave me feeling like I've made a good life decision, not a bad one. That's the thing – you can't be expected to continue a dieting plan that makes you feel hungry all of the time. I wouldn't expect you to, and neither would The Dash Diet. It is designed to let you take in smaller portions that make you feel like you had larger ones. That's a pretty good Jedi mind trick if there ever was one!

If you're like me, then you're probably not against eating healthier and shedding a few pounds. However, you're also not willing to change your entire concept of what it means to be alive and enjoy holidays, parties, and daily events. That's what I really like about The Dash Diet, you're able to maintain a healthier lifestyle, keep your blood pressure down, and improve your energy, all while you actually enjoy your meals. The Dash Diet is becoming increasingly popular, and for good reason – it works. It's not a particularly hard diet to follow because there are a lot of meals you can eat with the large variety of approved ingredients. Another huge benefit of The Dash Diet is that it's not overly expensive. You can find the allowable foods in almost any grocery store! If you're looking for a well-rounded way to reduce your weight, and improve your health, then you're in the right place.

THE SCIENCE BEHIND THE DASH DIET

The Dash Diet focuses on minimizing your sodium intake and increasing your consumption of nutrient rich foods. Originally developed out of studies sponsored by the National Institute of Health, it was initially designed to lower your cholesterol. However, over time it was shown to lessen your chances of heart disease, diabetes, blood pressure, cancer, and even promote a healthy heart. By reducing your consumption of sodium, saturated fats, and cholesterol, and increasing your intake of proteins, and healthy fats, your body reacts by leveling out your vitals. As we know, high amounts of sodium and trans fats not only increase your blood pressure, but also increase your risk of heart disease. Try not eating anything but bacon for a year and see how you feel – if you are even around anymore! Numerous studies done by the USDA, CDC, and many other institutions have shown that the average amount of nutrients (good and bad) that we wolf down are significantly higher than what a healthy person should be consuming. Why is that? There are a million and a half reasons, but the truth is that our daily habits are consistent with eating quick, fatty foods that are high in sodium. It's just a part of the American palette at this point. Imagine pouring a tablespoon of salt right into your mouth. What about a whole container of salt? That's pretty much what we do to our bodies every day. The Dash Diet was created to counteract that, and provide a fulfilling alternative by giving you foods low in sodium, and rich in health nutrients instead. Go figure that getting rid of the bad, and bringing in the good is beneficial!

Your body is almost always in one of two stages – fighting or feasting or feast or famine. You're fighting off bacteria, feasting on vitamins, fighting a disease, feasting on UV Rays, you're quite often doing one or two of those at the same time! Knowing that, the goal should be to do the right kind of feasting, so you don't have to do as much fighting. By eating healthier foods, you can let the food you consume do most of the work for you. That will relieve your blood pressure, become preventative in nature, and probably even lower your stress level. If you look at the way our metabolisms operate, then you'll know that you can't exactly eat one saltine cracker a day and be satisfied. As a matter of fact, because the human body processes foods at different speed levels, some of us are left feeling hungrier than others when our meals are gone. The Dash Diet provides a vast amount of ingredients for you to combine, that can amount to larger portions for higher metabolisms, and smaller portions for lower metabolisms.

In short, The Dash Diet is going to help you reduce your sodium intake, increase your digestion of healthy proteins, minimize your absorption of saturated fats and trans-fats, and fill you up with healthier alternatives that don't taste like cardboard. If you are used to dousing your food in salt, it might take a little longer to get used to, but you might just found that you enjoy the taste of food when it is natural.

HYPERTENSION AND THE DASH DIET

What you eat on a daily basis can help you lower your blood pressure and reduce your risk of stroke and heart disease.

When the Dietary Approaches to Stop Hypertension (DASH) diet started, it was just to stop the effects of high blood pressure by lowering it to a respectable level. Through the years, it has been shown to reduce blood pressure as well as put you back in a general state of better health.

According to the National Heart, Lung, and Blood Institute (NHLBI), your blood pressure can be unhealthy even if it stays only slightly above 120/80 mm Hg on a daily basis. Of course, you spike when you are stressed or when you eat badly for a day or two. However, the real problem comes when you exceed that on a daily basis. The higher you are above that level, the greater your health risk. Over time, high blood pressure makes your heart work too hard, which can cause stroke, hardening of the arteries, heart failure, kidney disease, and even blindness.

WHY THIS DIET WORKS

Why the DASH is a diet so effective at reducing blood pressure, you may ask.

It works because it combines many nutrients that have been shown to be beneficial in reducing blood pressure and inflammation within the body. Those nutrients include calcium, potassium, magnesium, protein, and fiber, as well as lower total fat and saturated fat.

The DASH diet is naturally lower in salt than is the typical American diet. The Dash diet recommends menus containing 2,300 mg of sodium and 1,500 mg of sodium a day, that means less than a tablespoon of salt per day. You can see someone putting more than that on their fries at a fast food restaurant!

It works so well, in fact, that following the DASH diet may delay your need to take hypertension medication, and may even keep you from needing to take it at all. And if you're already on medication, it may help you reduce the amount you take. It can also stop you from needing pricey, risky procedures that will require hospital stays, rehabilitation, and lifestyle changes.

Although the DASH diet isn't designed for weight loss, it can easily promote it if you reduce the number of servings you consume. Weight loss also lowers your blood pressure naturally. Losing just ten pounds can mean needing medication and not needing it! Most of the food that the diet features is low in energy density, which means it's big in volume and low in calories.

Moving Forward

If you decide to do The Dash Diet for your hypertension, adopt the DASH diet gradually. By doing so, you'll be more apt to stick to it long-term, breaking the habits that got you to the point you are currently at.

For example, add one more serving of vegetables at lunch and dinner if you eat only one or two servings a day now. You might also add fruit to meals and snacks if you now only have juice for breakfast. In addition, slowly increase your dairy products to three servings per day. Try drinking skim milk with lunch or dinner, instead of soda, alcohol, or tea.

WHAT RESULTS CAN I EXPECT?

Provided that you follow the Dash Diet for at least four weeks (one month), you should see significant results. Some of these will include improved energy, some weight loss, and better blood pressure. There have even been claims from losing 20lbs – 60lbs in six months! That's not a bad setup for merely changing how you eat what you eat.

Everyone is different, and people will experience different results, but with the acclamations and the success stories of The Dash Diet, it's hard to go wrong. Of course, it's not a terrible idea to combine some exercise with The Dash Diet, and you will experience results quicker. Start now, make it a habit. Transition if you have to, but the important (and cool) thing is that you can get going right now without cleaning out your cabinets or buying expensive machinery! The hardest thing about results from programs like these, is that they are usually not what you expected, and take too long to achieve. However with The Dash Diet, you should be able to experience noticeable results within the first month, as many people have. Take your blood pressure, step on that dreaded scale, and get your cholesterol checked.

Start The Dash Diet and stick with it religiously for one month. At the end of the month, when you excitedly step back on that scale, check your blood pressure, and get your cholesterol checked out, I'm confident you will be pleasantly surprised. Imagine what you could do if you did it for six months? For a year? Crazy.

Now here's the thing: You will get discouraged. Plan for that, because it's inevitable. When your friends are tearing up that foot long Coney, and you're sitting there with your tasty, healthy food, the thought of quitting will likely flash through your mind. So how do you combat that? Stay motivated. Join an online discussion board, hold yourself accountable, and most importantly, have someone else who can hold you accountable. Having someone who can encourage you, be disappointed I you when you fail, and help you pick yourself up is invaluable. Find a friend who can go on The Dash Diet with you! If you can keep it up, the results will start pouring in, and your peers (those Coney eating ones) will start saying "You've lost weight! What are you doing?" and that will be worth sacrificing for. In this technological age, there are even mobile apps that you can download that will keep you on track. Ultimately, your chances of living longer and spending less time (and money) in the hospital are much better. Not to mention you won't have to bunk up with those same friends in a nursing home when you're only 60. In the end, like everything in this world, The Dash Diet is what you make it. If you put your all into it, you'll see all the results. If you only put your half into it, you'll see half the results. So start today and reap the benefits!

THE MECHANINCS OF THE DASH DIET

So, all of this talk about what it does and how it works, now it's time to learn how to do it. According to the NHLBI*, your calorie intake works like this:

Daily Calorie Needs for Women

A quick rule of thumb is 10x current body weight.
Ex. If you weigh 150lb, you need 1500 calories to stay the same weight.

Daily Calorie Needs for Men

A quick rule of thumb is 11x current body weight.
Ex. If you weigh 190lb, you need 2090 calories to stay the same weight.

So once you've figured out where you are, you need to create a calorie deficit by diet and exercise to lose weight. Here's where The Dash Diet comes in: You need to figure your BMR using the method above (or calculate it more precisely online – search for 'calorie calculator'). Then find your closest number of calories across the top of the table below to find your recommended serving suggestions.

DASH Eating Plan—Number of Food Servings by Calorie Level

Food Group	1,200 Cal.	1,400 Cal.	1,600 Cal.	1,800 Cal.	2,000 Cal.	2,600 Cal.	3,100 Cal.
Grains[a]	4–5	5–6	6	6	6–8	10–11	12–13
Vegetables	3–4	3–4	3–4	4–5	4–5	5–6	6
Fruits	3–4	4	4	4–5	4–5	5–6	6
Fat-free or low-fat dairy products[b]	2–3	2–3	2–3	2–3	2–3	3	3–4
Lean meats, poultry, and fish	3 or less	3–4 or less	3–4 or less	6 or less	6 or less	6 or less	6–9
Nuts, seeds, and legumes	3 per week	3 per week	3–4 per week	4 per week	4–5 per week	1	1
Fats and oils[c]	1	1	2	2–3	2–3	3	4
Sweets and added sugars	3 or less per week	3 or less per week	3 or less per week	5 or less per week	5 or less per week	≤2	≤2
Maximum sodium limit[d]	2,300 mg/day	2,300 mg/day	2,300 mg/day	2,300 mg/day	2,300 mg/day	2,300 mg/day	2,300 mg/day

[a] Whole grains are recommended for most grain servings as a good source of fiber and nutrients.

[b] For lactose intolerance, try either lactase enzyme pills with dairy products or lactose-free or lactose-reduced milk.

[c] Fat content changes the serving amount of fats and oils. For example, 1 Tbsp regular salad dressing = one serving; 1 Tbsp low-fat dressing = one-half serving; 1 Tbsp fat-free dressing = zero servings.

[d] The DASH eating plan has a sodium limit of either 2,300 mg or 1,500 mg per day.

*https://www.nhlbi.nih.gov/health/health-topics/topics/dash/followdash.html

WHAT DOES THIS ALL MEAN?

So, this means you need to consume a lot of whole grains and vegetables. Start balancing your diet based on these tables, and you will start to see results. Notice the significance placed on limiting sodium consumption, in combination with your balance of the other food groups. One very popular method of attacking The Dash Diet is to go head first and cut out whole grains, fruits, cheese, and pretty much anything with sugar for the first 2 weeks. Then start introducing those back into your diet slowly in the third week. This is like joining The Polar Bear Club and diving into some ice water. This can be hard to maintain even for the first two weeks, so though it may be effective, is left up to your discretion.

Overall, this looks like:
(see below to see what fits into these categories)

Six to eight daily servings of grains and grain products, such as whole wheat bread, cereal, oatmeal, crackers, unsalted pretzels, and popcorn. A serving size is one slice of bread, one cup of ready-to-eat cereal, or a half-cup of rice, pasta, or cereal.

Four to five daily servings of vegetables — the darker in color, the better. A serving size is one cup of raw leafy vegetables, a half-cup of cooked vegetables, or six ounces of vegetable juice.

Four to five daily servings of fruit. A serving is one medium fruit, quarter-cup of dried fruit, half-cup of fresh, frozen or canned fruit, or six ounces of fruit juice.

Two or three daily servings of low-fat or fat-free dairy products. A serving is eight ounces of milk, one cup of yogurt, or 1½ ounces of cheese.

Six or fewer daily servings of lean meat, poultry, or fish. A serving is one ounce of cooked meats, skinless poultry, or fish.

Four to five servings per week of nuts, seeds, and dry beans. A serving is one-third cup or 1½ ounces of nuts, one tablespoon or half-ounce of seeds, or half-cup cooked dried beans.

Two to three small daily servings of fats and oils, such as olive oil and low-fat salad dressing. A serving is one teaspoon soft margarine, one tablespoon low-fat mayonnaise, two tablespoons light salad dressing, or one teaspoon vegetable oil.

Five or fewer servings per week of sweets, such as maple syrup, sorbet, or gelatin. A serving is one tablespoon sugar, one tablespoon jelly or jam, half-ounce jellybeans, or eight ounces of lemonade.

In the next chapter we will go over some ingredients and meal plans, so we are going to focus on properly managing these food groups. Your goal with The Dash Diet should be to reduce your portion size, increase your intake of healthy food groups, and most importantly, get creative. The tables above don't describe pouring a bunch of nuts, green stuff, and raw meat into a blender and drinking one shake per day. It is a guideline for your meals. One of the benefits of this is that you don't have to pay a lot of attention to calorie counting or other pesky numbers and symbols when you are purchasing your foods. What is important to you, is the quality of the foods you are eating, and keeping the ingredients standalone. What does that mean? That means no TV dinners, where everything is combined for you, and a bunch of MSG is mixed with heart attacks and clogged arteries.

That doesn't mean you have to spend all your time in the kitchen either, there are some really simple meal plans that can be made in little to no time that we will go over later. What you need to do is start thinking about what your daily meals look like right now. Are you hitting the McDonalds on the corner every day on your lunch break? Do you pack your lunches? Do you cook dinner, or do you sit down at a table to eat every evening? Grab a pen and paper and diagram your eating habits. This will be very useful in designing (and maintaining) your new strategy for a healthier lifestyle. It's absolutely essential that you know where, what, and how you're eating already so you can implement this revolutionary system. Once you have your meal schedules down, on another piece of paper, start ranking your food by healthy, unhealthy, healthier, and catastrophically dangerous to your health. This will allow you to transition slowly by replacing your more destructive meals with healthier alternatives based on the charts above. Or if you're gung-ho and want to dive head first, start replacing all your meals. The point is that you probably partake of foods you like, and satisfy you. By making this list, you will be able to compare your current eating system with your new one, and allow you to choose Dash Diet alternatives that are similar to what you're eating now. It's paramount that you start thinking in terms of your lifestyle, rather than your habits. It's hard to change a habit, but it's unbelievably difficult to change a lifestyle. That's what we are really talking about here, is it's time to overhaul your eating lifestyle. Most people don't start dieting with that in mind, and it's one of the reasons why it becomes so difficult. It's very easy to quit dieting, but it means something much more to quit a lifestyle.

How you proceed with The Dash Diet is entirely up to you, but if you want the recipe for success, it looks something like this:

You decide to begin The Dash Diet.
You commit.
You persevere.
You achieve results.
You commit.
You persevere.
You achieve results.

Notice the pattern? Making the decision is the first step, and congratulate yourself for doing so! After that begins, the incredible road of committing, persevering, and achieving starts, and you need to make sure you work your way through the steps. You see it's not just a hop on the bandwagon process, it's something that you have to continually strive for. That's what makes something like this difficult, most people don't grasp that it's a lifestyle. But you, you know it's a lifestyle. And knowing that will make the journey so much easier, and much more pleasant. You will be able to roll those sly comments right off your shoulders. You'll be able to look the other way when you see that Mushroom Swiss Burger that will give you a coronary artery disease. You'll be able to hold your head high, knowing that you've won. You've overcome temptations and rushed past roadblocks. There's no stopping you!

Now let's create your meal plans, and set you up for a healthier, better lifestyle!

FOODS TO EAT

Since you will be embarking on this new food schedule, it might be best to list some foods you're encouraged to eat in *limited amounts* on The DASH Diet Weight Loss Solution...

Dairy

Cheeses – low-fat or nonfat whole cheese or reduced fat / light cottage cheese. Examples: Laughing Cow Light Cheese Wedge, Mini Babybel Light, Kraft 2% Singles, light string cheese, 2% mozzarella.

Yogurt – unsweetened or artificially sweetened. Should be 120 calories or less for an 8-ounce serving or less than 100 calories for a 6-ounce serving

Nuts, beans, seeds

Nuts – preferably non-roasted and unsalted – e.g. almonds, cashews, peanuts, pistachios, walnuts.
Seeds e.g. sesame seeds

Peanut butter – natural, not reduced-fat (keep in the refrigerator and store upside down) or you can try PB2, which is powdered peanut butter that has a lot less fat and is natural.

Avocados are good, but try not to eat too many of them as they are high in fat. Consider adding them to a meal you have no good fats for.

Legumes

Beans e.g. black beans, kidney beans, Lentils, Soy foods.

Lean proteins

Choose a portion size about the size of your palm or the size of a deck of cards if you don't have a meat scale.

Lean meat examples include beef (broiled or roasted – top round, eye round, shoulder pot roast, round tip roast, shoulder steak, top sirloin steak, bottom round, top loin steak, tenderloin, t-bone, tri-tip, NY strip steak, ground beef 90% or 95% lean), pork (broiled or roasted – pork tenderloin, pork top loin roast, pork loin chop, pork center loin, pork sirloin, pork sirloin roast, Canadian bacon, lean ham, lean ground pork).

Lean poultry examples include chicken (roasted and skinless breast, thigh), turkey (skinless breast, whole, ground turkey with only white meat, no fat or skin)

Fish examples include anchovies, bluefish, catfish, cod, cod liver oil, flounder, haddock, halibut, herring, mackerel, ocean perch, orange roughy, oysters, pollock, rainbow trout, rockfish, salmon, sole, swordfish, tilapia, tuna canned in water, white fish

Shellfish (high quality)! Examples include blue crab, clams, lobster, scallops, shrimp – these are fine even though they are high in cholesterol, as they are very low in total fat and virtually free of saturated fat

Eggs – Egg substitutes and some whole eggs if desired. Choose eggs that are high in omega-3s

Heart-healthy fats!

Vegetable oils rich in monounsaturated fatty acid omega-3 like olive oil, canola oil, peanut oil, and other nut oils. Choose peanut oil for high-temperature cooking such as stir frying.

Foods that are especially rich in heart-healthy fats include avocados, nuts, seeds, olives, and many cold-water ocean fishes

Non-nutritive sweeteners

Sugar alcohols (e.g. sorbitol, mannitol, xylitol), other artificial sweeteners (e.g. Splenda, Truvia), natural non-caloric sweeteners (e.g. stevia).

While it has been popular to denigrate artificial sweeteners, they have a place in the diet for people who want to have sweet flavored foods but who can't handle the calories and/or sugar. Note that artificially sweetened baked goods and pastries are still high in starch and usually have calories equal to the original foods, which goes against this diet.

Other

Guacamole, Bouillon/broth (low-sodium), mustard, tomato paste, tomato sauce, vinegar, Worcestershire sauce, Fresh herbs including basil, bay leaves, cilantro, marjoram, oregano, parsley, rosemary, sage, thyme.

Spices including allspice, black pepper, cayenne pepper, chili powder, cinnamon, cumin, garlic powder, Italian seasoning, onion powder, paprika, poultry seasoning, salt substitutes, including lemon-pepper, Lemon juice, and lime juice

Vegetables

Cabbage, lettuce, onions, peas, eggplant, corn, spinach, sweet potatoes, blue potatoes, tomatoes, carrots, squash, zucchini, cucumber, and kale.

Fruits

Apples, oranges, mangoes, raisins, grapes, cherries, bananas, strawberries, blueberries, blackberries, raspberries, plums, pears, figs, pineapples, coconut, oranges, tangerines, and peaches.

Grains

Breads: whole wheat, pita, tortilla and grains like wild rice, couscous, quinoa, oats, whole wheat pasta, brown rice, and barley.

Foods to eat unlimited in general on The DASH Diet

While it wouldn't be great to eat these constantly every day, these are the foods you should keep around when you are hungry for snacks. Don't feel guilty about these!

Non-starchy vegetables

Examples include asparagus, beets, broccoli, brussels sprouts, cabbage, red cabbage, carrots, cauliflower, celery, cucumber, garlic, green beans/haricots verts, greens, jalapeño peppers and other hot peppers, jicama, lettuces, onions, peas, peppers, radishes, shallots, snow peas, spaghetti squash, sugar snap peas, summer squash, tomatoes, water chestnuts, zucchini

Feel free to munch on carrots and tomatoes, which are often unnecessarily avoided in low-carb plans. Coleslaw is a superfood when it comes to The Dash Diet.

Beverages

Many people often don't think about the calories they consume when they are drinking. Also, hunger pangs are often associated with dehydration rather than hunger. If you feel hungry, try to drink a glass of water before you chow down on something else.

Water, Black coffee. (use only non-caloric sweeteners), unsweetened or artificially sweetened tea, diet sodas, sugar-free Vegetable juices such as tomato juice, V8 juice – low sodium.

FOODS TO AVOID

These are the foods that, in general, you should try to stay away from. Once again, it is okay to treat yourself, but limit these foods to once a week or so. It may be handy to keep this as a cheat sheet to glance at before you eat something questionable until it's natural.

- Salt
- Alcohol (keep this to a minimum)
- Fats – Saturated, trans-fats
- Processed meat
- Frozen foods/TV Dinners
- Sodas
- Chinese food (high in sodium)
- Canned soups & fruits
- Pickles (high in sodium)
- Fast Food (obviously)
- Bacon (high in sodium, keep it to a minimum)
- Donuts
- Candy/Chocolate Bars
- Soy Sauce
- Bouillon Cubes
- Yeast Extract
- Pretzels
- Popcorn
- Pizza
- Cheese (minimum)

- Canned Tuna
- Whipped Cream
- Coffee (reduce consumption)
- Dark Chocolate
- Butter (minimum)

RECIPE IDEAS

So what would an average meal look like? This is where you get to be creative. Start mixing and matching ingredients, and keep in mind the lists above aren't all inclusive. There are lots of foods out there that will fit The Dash Diet bill. Here are some quick examples to get you going.

Breakfast Ideas

- 1 Whole Wheat Bagel – W/ no salt peanut butter
- 1 orange
- 1 cup of coffee w/ fat free milk

- 1 Bowl Oatmeal w/ blueberries
- 1 cup of low-fat yogurt
- 1 Low-fat Yogurt based Strawberry smoothie

- 2 Egg Omelets
- 1 Wheat Toast
- Spinach topped w/ bits of sunflower seeds & 1 teaspoon olive oil

Lunch Ideas

- 1 Bowl Couscous
- 1 Side Serving of Lentils w/ Tomatoes
- 1 Cup of Mango

———————

- 1 Chicken Breast topped with Rosemary & Lemmon Pepper
- 1 Side salad drizzled w/ teaspoon of olive oil & 1 teaspoon raisins

———————

- 1 Fruit Bowl – Think blueberries, Strawberries, Pears, Pineapples
- 1 Low-Fat Yogurt
- 1 Smoothie

Dinner Ideas

- 1 Baked Tilapia Topped with Green Beans, Thyme, and Freshly Squeezed Lemon Juice
- 1 Side of Roasted Bell Peppers, Sun Dried Tomatoes, and Asparagus

———————

- 1 Serving Cubed Baked Potato Slices, Mixed with Olive Oil, Mushrooms, and Curried Chicken
- 1 Side of Romaine Lettuce Salad Topped with Olive Oil and Dates

———————

- 1 Serving Whole Wheat Pasta w/ Spaghetti Sauce
- 1 Lightly Toasted Garlic Whole Wheat Bread

GLUTEN-FREE AND DAIRY-FREE
ALTERNATIVES

The most common food allergens people run into problems with when they are trying The Dash Diet are wheat (gluten or Celiac), peanuts and tree nuts, dairy (cow's milk), fish and shellfish, soy, and eggs. Since dairy and nuts are part of the key foods for the DASH Diet and a well-balanced diet overall, here are ways around the allergens / sensitivities.

Dairy sensitivities

Allergy or sensitivity to cow's milk: Consider trying goat's milk products and other non-cow-sourced dairy foods if you can tolerate them. If not, follow your doctor's or dietitian's advice regarding dairy. Only do this if you are truly allergic to cow's milk, however.

Lactose intolerance: Many people find that they can consume all dairy foods if they add Lactaid drops to their milk or use Lactaid milk. Others might be able to use acidophilus milk without having any symptoms

Nondairy substitutes are fine, but not preferred: make sure that they have similar calcium and vitamin D levels as the dairy foods they replace. Avoid those products that are highly sweetened or "flavored" as that usually means added salt, sugar, or chemicals.

Nut allergies

Try avocados as a great substitute, as they have similar nutrients to nuts You can also forget about nuts and get your healthy fats from olive oil and/or fatty fish. You may need to have a few extra servings of fruits and veggies to be sure you are getting enough potassium

Gluten sensitivity or true celiac disease

Many options listen above (quinoa, couscous, etc) are gluten free.

Other types of food allergies

(eggs, seafood, beans, etc)
Make substitutions with foods having similar nutrients.

If you have more complicated allergies or other food digestive issues, you may want to consult with a dietitian to adapt the DASH diet for your personal needs.

STAYING MOTIVATED AND AVOIDING PITFALLS

As you can see, The Dash Diet isn't terribly difficult to follow, and its benefits are quite vast. However, that doesn't mean it's easy to maintain without a little work on your part. It's not just the times when you're with your friends or family that you have to be careful, it's when you're by yourself or when you're bored. It will be difficult at first, but you have to commit! After all, nothing comes easy, or free. Keeping a healthy diet is more than what you put in your mouth, it's what you put in your mind that might be even more important. Keeping a proper mental attitude about yourself is what will ultimately lead to your success with The Dash Diet. This rings true of any endeavor, whether it's business, personal or any achievement you have ever made, it didn't come without sacrifice, and hard work. The hard work that you have to put into The Dash Diet will feed your ability to conquer your mental roadblocks. These roadblocks will come in all shapes and sizes, and will come from different angles every day! You have to prepare yourself for the expected hindrances, Thanksgiving dinners, Christmas dinners, the fast food joint on your way home from work, all of these will temp you. You need to have a strong will, and a strong mind to defeat these obstacles, but how do you do that? You train yourself to accept nothing but success!

There is no negotiating, there is no "Maybe just this once..." no excuses, and, most importantly, no failure! You have to think in terms of the here and now, and the future. Everyone wants to be happy with their health, size, and their confidence level. That's something you can achieve with a fit body, mind, and soul. Begin now by saying to yourself "I won't quit, I won't lose, and I won't stop." Your mind is the most powerful tool, and it will help you accomplish anything you desire. If what you want is a truly healthy lifestyle, to live long and prosper so to speak, then you have to learn how to overcome the hard times, as well as celebrate the good times. Disregard what people say about your new way of eating, don't listen to naysayers, focus on you, and how you want to feel. In the end, people will always have an opinion about your choices, but the most important opinion of all, is yours. That's why surrounding yourself with like-minded people will help you succeed with The Dash Diet. There are a lot of tricks you can use, to keep your mind steady on what is important. One of those, as we have discussed, is staying in touch with support groups, and being around the people who are where you want to be. Another is subliminal, tricking your mind into doing exactly what you want.

This method requires minimal effort, is creative in nature, and anyone can do it! Leave notes for yourself in the fridge, in your pantry, on your nightstand – wherever you may be tempted the most! Leave encouraging notes in your car, on your desk at work, make it your wallpaper on your computer. Set alarms on your phone at breakfast, lunch and dinner to remind you of your goals. Keep a small chalkboard in your kitchen with your objectives on it. Purchase index cards, and write down congratulations for achieving milestones, and give them to yourself in the future when you accomplish them! There's no end to all of the imaginative ways you can remind yourself, uplift yourself, celebrate with yourself, and stay on the right path. Many people begin diet plans and exercising routines quickly, and stray from them even quicker. If you want to utilize The Dash Diet for your lifestyle, then you have to commit to it! You have to repeat those words, "I won't quit, I won't lose, and I won't stop." Say them every day, and never forget them. That is your new mantra. It may seem silly, but it works. All you have to do is put in the effort. We talked about this before - that nothing comes easy or free, and having mentioned that in passing, it's time to really pay attention to what that means.

The Dash Diet is a state of mind, that you are going to live a healthier life, and you're going to love it! Diets don't have to be boring, time-consuming, expensive methods that take too much work. They can be exciting, fun, and worthwhile. The most important thing for you to remember is how thankful you will be when you are looking back over your life, and you see the good choices you made. This is one of those choices that will let you see your grandkids grow up. You won't have to worry about those massive hospital bills, and you won't have to have that conversation with yourself. You know which one, the conversation that goes something like "I should have taken better care of myself." That alone is worth every cent and sweat you put into The Dash Diet. The choices you make now are changing your future. Start making the right choices, and you'll have a better future! There are a lot of tough decisions you have made, and will have to continue to make. That will never end, as it is a part of life's grand design. One thing is certain, and that is the fact that your eating habits are an infinitesimally small factor in your life. Sure, eating Fast Food all the time is fun and tasty, but the future you, will tell your younger self that it isn't worth it. All the greasy, fat, menacing foods that tear your stomach apart now will tear your arteries apart later. You can change this factor in your life. A small change, with incredible results. All you have to do is start.

Finally, here are some last minute tips to help you stay on track, lose weight, and get healthier with The DASH Diet.

- Do not skip over any meals or snacks just because you want to lose more weight. If you find that you are getting hungry shortly after meals, then your serving sizes are too small, especially the protein part
- Have a good balance of bulky, filling foods (e.g. vegetables) along with protein-rich foods
- Make half your plate nonstarchy veggies! (Super important!)
- If you start to feel a little light-headed or dizzy, have another snack (or make sure you had the snack in the first place)
- Don't be overly restrictive with salts.
- Focus on making your plate colorful – e.g. salads should have more than just green lettuce
- Try a food bare before you add any seasonings to it – you will be surprised at how good some foods are naturally.
- Get plenty of fluids, at least 8 glasses per day – be careful of overdrinking water though, as that can lead to problems with your sodium levels – you can actually get very sick from having too much water!
- Caffeinated beverages, other liquids, and water that comes from foods (including fruits, vegetables, and jello) all count towards this. Drinking water with meals does almost nothing to quench hunger, but eating foods that are high in water content, including (low-sodium) soups, fruits, and vegetables, helps you avoid overeating

Choose foods that you like and don't be afraid to treat yourself every once in a while. You will never succeed if you are too rigid.

CONCLUSION

I want to personally Thank You again for picking up a copy of this book!

Ultimately The Dash Diet is what you make it. It's been a common theme in this book that how you approach and maintain The Dash Diet will directly correlate with the results you see. All you have to do is manage your foods properly, be creative, and have a steady mind. If you can do those things, then The Dash Diet will work for you! Lucky for you, The Dash Diet has worked for many other people, and it can also work to your benefit as well. You have everything you need to get started right now, inside you. As a matter of fact, the only thing that's holding you back is yourself! Start putting together all the reasons why you should start today, and ask yourself why you haven't started already? If it's something you've always wanted to do, then go for it! In my experience, it is always the people that start early, that finish strong. With hard work, effort and determination, you can achieve absolutely anything, including this! Why not you? That's a question that I have heard before, that rings through my head every time I think of it. Why not me? Why not you? There's absolutely nothing in your way but yourself, and that even that can be a hard bridge to cross. But keep your mind steady, your plate full, and your commitment high, and you will have the success you want from The Dash Diet! Most importantly you want to focus on the future, more than the here and now. Pay attention to the life you expect to live because that picture is the one you need to paint. The Dash Diet can work for anyone who sets their mind to practicing it. There's not a person that it can't work for, and that includes you. There are no excuses, no failures, only success. In the end, The Dash Diet is an incredibly well-rounded dietary planning system that can keep your weight loss down, as well as your blood pressure. As stated in the beginning, those aren't the only benefits, including reduced risk of cancer, but also kidney disease, diabetes, heart failure, stroke, improved energy, and most importantly – A sound mind. Because that's what we are all really after, peace of mind.

After all, that's what we all really want, to know that we have made the right decisions in life, and to keep doing so. The Dash diet is one of those right decisions, and it promotes health benefits, as well as mental benefits. It takes structure, responsibility, and accountability. Those are traits that are all too often forgotten, and they need to be remembered. Remind yourself, that you can achieve anything, and that nothing can hold you back except you. And most importantly, when you start to see results, encourage others to do the same! What good is The Dash Diet to you, if you have success with it and don't share it with others? Don't rob your friends and family of the advantages of this lifestyle, share it with them! Share it with your parents, your friends, your spouse, and your siblings. They will be forever grateful, and if they achieve success you will have the greatest feeling of all – gratitude. Manage your meals, and manage your health. The small steps you are required to take with The Dash Diet will provide you with a sound, peace of mind that you cannot describe in words. "I won't quit, I won't lose, and I won't stop."

So what are you waiting for?!

Finally, if you enjoyed this book, please take the time to share your thoughts and post a positive review on Amazon. I would greatly appreciate your support!

Thank you and good luck!

Benjamin Tideas

COPYRIGHT NOTICE

ADDITIONAL RESOURCES

Please point your web browser to
www.plaid-enterprises.com/dash-diet
for more resources, my full bibliography and to grab your FREE book!

Finally, I hope you enjoy the recipes that follow!

BONUS: DASH DIET RECIPES

Following are just a few recipes, adapted from the Mayo Clinic, for every part of your day that will help you vary your food choices, but still stick to the Dash Diet. Enjoy!!!

CRISPY POTATO SKINS

Ingredients

2 medium russet potatoes
Butter-flavored cooking spray
1 tablespoon minced fresh rosemary
1/8 teaspoon freshly ground black pepper

Directions

Preheat the oven to 375 F.

Wash potatoes and pierce with a fork. Bake until the skins are crisp, about 1 hour.

Carefully cut the potatoes in half and scoop out the pulp, leaving about 1/8 inch of the potato flesh attached to the skin. Save the pulp for another use.

Spray the inside of each potato skin with butter-flavored cooking spray. Press in the rosemary and pepper. Return the skins to the oven for 5 to 10 minutes. Serve immediately.

SHRIMP AND LIME SAUCE

Ingredients

1 medium red onion, chopped
1/2 cup fresh lime juice, plus lime zest as garnish
2 tablespoons capers
2 tablespoons Dijon mustard
1/2 teaspoon hot sauce
1 cup water
1/2 cup rice vinegar
3 whole cloves
1 bay leaf
1 pound uncooked shrimp, peeled and deveined

Directions

In a shallow baking dish, combine the onion, lime juice, capers, mustard and hot sauce. Set aside.

In a large saucepan, add the water, vinegar, cloves and bay leaf. Bring to a boil and add the shrimp.

Cook for 1 minute, constantly stirring .

Drain and transfer the shrimp to the shallow dish containing the onion mixture, making sure to discard the cloves and bay leaf. Stir to combine.

Cover and refrigerate until well chilled, about 1 hour.

To serve, divide the shrimp mixture among individual small bowls and garnish each with lime zest. Serve cold

GREEN SMOOTHIE

Ingredients

*3-4 services
1 banana
1/2 cup strawberries
Juice of 1 lemon (about 4 tablespoons)
1/2 cup other berries such as blackberries or blueberries
2 ounces fresh raw baby spinach (about 2 cups)
1 tablespoon fresh mint or to taste
1 cup cold water or ice

Directions

Place all ingredients in a blender or juicer and puree. Enjoy.

GOOD MORNING MOJITO

Ingredients

1/2 cup dark honey
1/2 cup fresh lime juice
1/2 cup firmly packed fresh mint leaves
2 cups fresh grapefruit juice, chilled
2 cups fresh orange juice, chilled
2 teaspoons grated lime zest
1 lime, cut into 6 slices

Directions

In a small saucepan, combine the honey and lime juice. Bring to a boil over medium heat.

Add the mint leaves and remove from the heat.

Steep the honey mixture for 5-7 minutes, then pass the mixture through a fine-mesh sieve placed over a bowl, pressing down lightly on the leaves with the back of a wooden spoon.

Refrigerate the syrup until cold.

In a large pitcher, combine the mint syrup, grapefruit and orange juices, and lime zest. Stir until the syrup is dissolved.

Pour into tall, chilled glasses and garnish each glass with a lime slice.

CHILI

Ingredients

1 pound extra-lean ground beef
1/2 cup chopped onion
2 large tomatoes (or 2 cups canned, unsalted tomatoes)
4 cups canned kidney beans, rinsed and drained
1 cup chopped celery
1 teaspoon sugar
1 1/2 tablespoons chili powder or to taste
Water, as desired
2 tablespoons cornmeal
Jalapeno peppers, seeded and chopped, as desired

Directions

In a soup pot, add the ground beef and onion. Over medium heat saute until the meat is browned and the onion is translucent. Drain well.

Add the tomatoes, kidney beans, celery, sugar and chili powder to the ground beef mixture.

Cover and cook for 10 minutes, frequently stirring.

Uncover and add water to desired consistency. Stir in cornmeal.

Cook for at least 10 minutes more to allow the flavors to blend.

Ladle into warmed bowls and garnish with jalapeno peppers, if desired. Serve immediately.

MANGO SALSA PIZZA

Ingredients

1 cup chopped red or green bell peppers
1/2 cup minced onion
1/2 cup mango, seeded, peeled and chopped
1/2 cup pineapple tidbits
1 tablespoon lime juice
1/2 cup fresh cilantro, chopped
1 12-inch prepared whole-grain pizza crust, purchased or made from a mix

Directions

Preheat the oven to 425 F. Lightly coat a 12-inch round baking pan with cooking spray.

In a small bowl, mix together the peppers, onions, mango, pineapple, lime juice and cilantro. Set aside.

Roll out dough and press into the baking pan. Place in the oven and cook about 15 minutes.

Take the pizza crust out of the oven and spread with mango salsa. Place the pizza back into the oven and bake until the toppings are hot and the crust is browned, about 5 to 10 minutes.

Cut the pizza into 8 even slices and serve immediately.

GRILLED ANGEL FOOD CAKE

Ingredients

1 1/2 cup strawberries, chopped
3/4 cup chopped rhubarb
1/2 cup sugar
6 tablespoons water
1 3/4 teaspoons vanilla
1/8 teaspoon cinnamon
1 prepared angel food cake, cut into 6 pieces
3/4 cup reduced-fat whipped topping

Directions

Prepare a hot fire in a charcoal grill or heat a gas grill or broiler. Away from the heat source, lightly coat the grill rack or broiler pan with cooking spray. Position the cooking rack 4 to 6 inches from the heat source.

To make the sauce, in a saucepan, combine the strawberries, rhubarb, sugar, water, vanilla and cinnamon.

Cook on medium heat until the mixture just starts to boil, about 5 minutes. Remove the saucepan from the heat and set aside.

Place the angel food cake toward the edge of the grill rack where there is less heat or on the broiler pan. Grill or broil until each side turns brown, about 1 to 3 minutes.

Place the angel food cake on individual serving plates. Top each piece with 1/4 cup of the strawberry-rhubarb sauce and 2 tablespoons of the whipped topping. Serve immediately.

RAINBOW ICE POPS

Ingredients

1 1/2 cups diced strawberries, **cantaloupe** and watermelon
1/2 cup blueberries
2 cups 100 percent apple juice (or another favorite juice)
6 paper cups (6-8 ounces each)
6 craft sticks

Directions:

Mix the fruit together and divide evenly into the paper cups. Pour 1/3 cup of juice into each paper cup.

Place the cups on a level surface in the freezer. Freeze until partially frozen, approximately 1 hour.

Insert craft stick into center of each pop.

Freeze until firm.